The Natural Cure For Smoking

ow The Magic Mineral Prevents The Desire To Smoke

Anthony Shkreli

The Natural Cure For Smoking
How The Magic Mineral Prevents The Desire To Smoke

Copyright © 2012
by Anthony Shkreli

ISBN: 978-0-9851353-4-8

Published by: Paracelsus Press

Imprint of
Seven Pillars House Publishing

Web-Site
www.smoking-is-hunger.com

For Barbara

Table Of Contents

Cave-Dwellers

If you are a smoker— it is not your fault. Because you are not addicted to nicotine . . .

In fact there is no such thing as nicotine or tobacco addiction. It is myth. It is on a par with old wives tales.

Ever heard that before?

And how about this one? The reason you smoke is because you are starving . . .

I'll bet you DEFINITELY have not heard that before. But sometimes when the truth is heard it can seem shocking because if the philosopher Plato is correct, we all just might be living in the proverbial cave. The shadows on the cave wall are not the substance or the reality, though mankind mistakenly takes those images for what is true.

The truth lies outside the cave, where the sun is shining. It may take a little bit to get our eyes adjusted to that bright sunshine, it comes as a shock to our system, because we are not accustomed to the light— the truth.

Its a little like this book. When you understand the ideas and principles set forth in this little book, and apply them, you will see things clearly and you may begin to resent all those false images and shadows that you were paying attention to before. This is only natural because what is revealed herein has never been heard before but it is the substance, it is the truth.

The natural thing to do, if you have been living in that cave of ignorance, would have been to shut off when I stated on the previous page that the reason you are smoking is because you are starving. What is this joker talking about?— you might have said this under your breath. But if you made it to this second page you just might have a chance to escape the cave.

Not many of you may know that there are two types of starvation. We are all familiar with the first type. But this book introduces the second type of hunger that has been known by scientists in the 20th century, like Curt Richter and Leslie Harris, which they called special-hunger. It is called special hunger because the body is starving for a **specific** nutrient. In other words, you may be eating plenty of food but the food may not contain a certain element which your cells need for proper functioning. So you become deficient in that nutrient.

And here is the strange thing that these scientists noted when a biological organism undergoes specific hunger: The organism does not take this deficiency lying down— it will not stand for this condition of lack.

The biological organism will actually seek out this 'missing' nutrient to try to maintain equilibrium and *it will even eat non-foods in order to do this*.

The consumption of non-foods by humans is a his-

3

torical fact. This condition is known in the medical community as *pica.*

People have been known to consume quite strange things like clay, glass, nails, laundry starch etc.—-even to this day. And it is not because there is no food available. However, what has been missed and overlooked by everyone is the fact that smokers are also consuming a non-food, though it is smoked. So why are they doing this?

Smokers and everyone else engaging in pica are deficient in a single nutrient. It is not available in the normal food supply (for various reasons which are more fully explained in my first book) so they must seek it in non-food forms.

If you are a smoker this is what you are suffering— a deficiency of one nutrient.

This is the concept and theoretical underpinning of this book and my previous one, **You Are Not Ad-**

dicted To Cigarette Smoking You Are Starving. But theories are only as good as their practicality—that is, does it work? In other words, if a person smokes because they are suffering from a nutrient deficiency that could only mean one thing . . .

If you replace the nutrient through diet, then the deficiency will go away. This means the cravings for non-food items, like tobacco, will also go away. The desire to smoke will vanish

This book is a summary, though with some added material, of my first book. I recommend reading the first book because it explains the science in detail. But if you just want the answer and a broad overview of the principles involved, this book packs a punch. Prepare yourself for some bright sunshine as you make your way out of the cave . . .

1 Hunting For Big-Foot

There is something very wrong with this picture. In the year 2000 at the 11th World Conference on Tobacco or Health in Chicago, the Surgeon General released a report on "Reducing Tobacco Use". One of the actions proposed to reduce tobacco use was to "encourage widespread use of state-of-the-art treatment of nicotine addiction." Along with a "combination of behavioral counseling and pharmacological treatment" the smoking epidemic would be mitigated. The green light was given for nicotine replacement therapies. Choose your weapon— patches, gums, inhalers and such would halt the tide of the nicotine addiction.

Flash forward to January of 2012 and we read the opening sentence of a press release from the Harvard School of Public Health: "Nicotine replacement therapies (NRTs) designed to help people stop smoking, specifically nicotine patches and nicotine gum, do not appear to be effective in helping smokers quit long-term, even when combined with smoking cessation counseling, according to a new study by researchers at Harvard School of Public Health (HSPH) and the University of Massachusetts Boston."

From no less than Dr. Michael Siegel, a physician and professor at Boston University's School of Public Health, we hear the following: "The levels of long-term success are dismal. More importantly, I think that the role of nicotine replacement therapy as part of a national policy to address smoking cessation has been over emphasized." This is a topic near and dear to Mr.Siegel who served as an expert witness in a lawsuit worth over $100 billion dollars against the tobacco companies . . . at least he's being honest.

Studies, and meta-studies of those same studies, show the same pattern— nicotine is not the addictive factor in cigarette smoking.

The facts are glaring and there are some professionals within the field that are breaking ranks— or saving face.

Professor Peter Killeen of Arizona State University is one of the first straws that are beginning to pile up on the camels back. In September of 2009 he gave a talk to present his research findings for the National Institute On Drug Abuse. The title of his talk? "Reefer Madness: There ain't no such Thing as Addiction to Nicotine"

According to Killeen, "Studies have shown that none of the nicotine replacement therapies — chewing gum, inhalers, patches — none of those are addictive. Nicotine is not addictive. So what's going on?"

He also added that, "Not everybody knows that nicotine is not addictive," he said. "This negatively affects both the research and public opinion."

Killeen is not only taking it to the streets but he is also presenting his findings to the starched intelligentsia: "I presented this position to 20 of the world's experts," he said. "And though some were shocked and insulted, no one could argue that my case was untrue."

We'll echo Killen's words . . . "What's going on?"

Killeen believes there is something missing in the whole equation of cigarette smoking— some missing factor. "It is my hypothesis that it's a combination of nicotine with some of these other chemicals that causes the powerful addiction."

Killeen is only repeating what has been found in laboratories across the world. He is only a spokesman trying to bring everyone up to speed. Its astonishing that the public does not know this about cigarettes but it seems that the gatekeepers have been effective in keeping it secret.

Killeen calls this missing factor, along with nicotine, 'the one-two punch.' The combination of this missing factor with nicotine is what causes the so-called addiction. Nicotine by itself is not the cause.

This missing factor is doing something in the brain that is very efficient and effective but it is only leaving footprints behind. Like Big-Foot, no one has really captured this elusive substance. That this missing factor has been responsible for this certain action in the brain has been known since at least 1993.

Meanwhile back at the ranch the so-called health authorities were pushing nicotine replacement on everyone.

Since nicotine is not the addictive factor by itself, what is this mysterious missing factor that is part of the one-two punch that keeps smokers coming back for that cigarette?

2 Smoking Is Hunger

Curt Richter found out some quite amazing things. If there is an underrated scientist of the 20th century it is Curt Richter. The man was tireless. All he did was plug away in his laboratory for most of his life and publish scientifice papers in such diverse fields as neurology, endocrinology, psychology and physiology.

But even more than that, Curt Richter (though he has passed on) and his voluminous research are going to help us solve one of the great mysteries of the last 100 or so years— what is causing people to smoke?

This means he is going to shed some special light on that so-called 'missing factor' in tobacco.

In one of his many areas of research Richter discovered, through countless and rigorous experiments, a rather strange phenomenon. He came to call this phenomenon 'self-selection' ---the implications of this discovery are so far reaching that it even touches upon the seemingly unrelated field of tobacco addiction.

For many years, since the time of the scientist Claude Bernard there was one central understanding about the human body and it was this: Whenever the body becomes out of balance due to some stressor, the body responds to this imbalance by correcting it— by bringing balance.

How does it do this? There are many mechanisms that the body unleashes to bring everything back into balance but the central point must be understood and grasped:

The body seeks to bring back balance whenever there is imbalance. The fancy name for this is home-ostasis (*homeo*-same *stasis*-state). The body seeks to keep things at an even keel— a steady state.

A simple example of this is the brain. It needs fuel . . . but it needs this fuel all the time.

But here is the problem— you are not eating all the time and the brain needs glucose all the time so---

How does the body solve this potential problem, this imbalance?

It releases stored glucose from the liver during those times you are not eating. This ensures a steady supply of fuel to the brain to keep things at a steady state— homeostasis.

So we could say that the body has internal mechanisms to keep things flowing smoothly in the inside. The body, we could say, is self-regulating.

What does this have to do with cigarette smoking? Everything, as we shall see . . .

Richter's genius lies in the fact that he noticed, through animal studies, that the body has a way of regulating the interior environment through external actions. In other words, if there is some type of internal imbalance the organism will seek to balance the distortion through external actions by selecting a food or even a non-food to correct the imbalance inside.

An easy example of this is the thing known as hunger— we've all felt it. What is this really? It is actually an imbalance and the body is signalling us to correct it or else. The cells need nutrients to carry out their functions. Its real simple— if they don't we die.

So through an external action we correct the imbalance by eating and thereby giving those cells the materials they need to function. An external action corrects an internal imbalance.

Richter took his cue from this state called hunger and this is where his genius came shining through. Scientists even before Richter came to discover that there was another type of hunger which you may not be familiar with.

Scientists at the time called this hunger— *special* hunger. This is hunger for a *specific* nutrient— one nutrient— and scientists refer to this as a deficiency. It can be any nutrient and the deficiency can happen for many reasons. Poor diet selection, geographical location or food processing may remove the nutrient. If this deficiency occurs for a long period of time, scientists realize that this can cause disease.

But here is where it gets weird. In the laboratory, Richter created *artificial* deficiencies of certain nutrients— he purposely withheld certain nutrients from the diet of the rats.

For example, in one study which was published in the journal Science in 1937 (86:354), Richter removed thiamine or vitamin B-1 from the diets of rats. Soon after the deficiency was established, Richter then provided 13 containers of foods in solution, being very careful to make sure that there was no thiamine in any of the containers— except for one container.

Here is the weird part. The rats invariably chose

15

the container with thiamine in it, disregarding the others. In fact, Richter reported that the rats were so greedy for the thiamine bottle that when attempts were made to remove the thiamine filled bottle, the rats clung to the bottle with claws and teeth.

How did the rats distinguish one nutrient from all the other food stuffs? Somehow the rats were able to *select* thiamine from their environment to correct their thiamine imbalance.

This strange ability to detect the 'missing factor' to correct an imbalance Richter called *self-selection*. That is, the organism selects a food item in order to correct an imbalance.

Richter also demonstrated this principle by creating an imbalance in the rat using surgical techniques. For example in one experiment he removed the adrenal glands in the rats. Normally rats would die within about a week of this operation on a normal diet because the adrenals are responsible for salt metabolism— the organism will not be able to retain any sodium which is necessary in most cellular functions.

But when given free access to a salt solution the rats *selected* this solution and drank freely from it and lived! The internal imbalance–the adrenals removed–was corrected by the external action of the rats.

When Richter removed the parathyroid from rats he found the same same principle operating. The parathyroid is the calcium manager of the body. Its job is to maintain constant levels of free ionized calcium in the blood. If there are extreme deficits of calcium intake the parathyroid will actually attack bone strcture to release calcium into the blood supply. But what happens when you remove it? The manager is gone and not able to correct the imbalance inside.

But the astounding thing Richter found was that

when given free access to a calcium solution these rats freely selected this whenever they needed it. They were correcting the imbalance created by the surgical removal of the parathyroid. Again, we see an external action correcting an interior imbalance.

Could it be that the cigarette smoker is selecting something in his environment (tobacco) to correct an interior imbalance? Does that mean that tobacco contains a nutrient that the cigarette smoker is lacking? But tobacco isn't a food . . .

Here is Richters genius again to show us a vital principle. The strange thing about to be unveiled for us by Richter can be summed up in this way:

To correct an imbalance an organism will seek a missing nutrient or missing factor even if it is in a non-food . . .

Make sure you read the last sentence again before proceeding.

Because here is what Richter found in another experiment. He deprived rats of the B family of vitamins for a period of time. During the whole experiment the rats always had plenty of food— the only thing was none of the food contained B complex. Now for the weird part.

Richter then presented rat dung from healthy rats into the cages. Normally the rats didn't eat dung when they had a balanced diet. But these rats attacked that poop like there was no tomorrow, rather than eat the food in their cage. What was going on?

It was the principle of self-selection all over again. How could this be? Well, it is an established fact that the colon, through microbacteria, produces the B family of vitamins. The rats were eating a non-food because it was carrying something that corrected their inner deficiency of the B complex vitamins.

To correct an imbalance an organism will seek a

19

missing nutrient or missing factor even if it is in a non-food.

This is exactly what is occurring in cigarette smoking. If we can find what that missing factor is then the smoking problem is solved.

Let's put it this way. The rats in that previous experiment would have stopped eating the non-food, the dung, if they had been presented with a food that contained B complex.

But the same should go for the smoker. If the smoker is presented with that 'missing factor' through his diet then they will not want the non-food— tobacco. Its as simple as that. All we need to do is identify what it is that the tobacco plant is carrying that is lacking in our modern diet and the smokng problem is solved.

In the next chapter the 'missing factor' is unveiled but what is interesting is that it has been known about for thousands of years. It hasn't been easy to identify because the ancient Indians veiled it in myth . . .

3

My Brother Tobacco

The strange thing about the 'missing factor' is that it is sort of hidden— but not completely. What is interesting is that modern science will help the missing factor come out into the light. But first we must see where it is hidden.

In the ancient Indian tradition there are many myths about the origin and the nature of tobacco. The myths that talk about the nature of tobacco are very interesting because they seem to point to:

1) properties of tobacco and

2) the composition of tobacco

If we can interpret these specific areas of the myths with the help of modern science, then we may be able to identify the missing factor that is making people smoke.

According to the Indians, at one point in time, mankind turned to evil and this Fall of man had an effect upon nature. The plant, animal and rock kingdoms decided to hold a conference to deal with this new evil order of things. The Bear tribe represented the animal kingdom and they proposed a plan to lessen the evil in the world. "We must shorten man's life on the earth. If men are allowed to live long lives then they will bring destruction to the earth."

Their plan to do this? " We will introduce disease into the world."

The other two tribes reluctantly agreed but the plant tribe had pity upon man and spoke up louder than the rest. Now the plant tribe was represented by none other than— *tobacco*. And tobacco wanted to make mans life a little easier amongst all the disease that man would soon face so tobacco spoke up and said, " I will be the sacred herb and help people to return to the sacred life." Tobacco, being head of the plant kingdom, appointed various plants to help ease the pain of man's suffering. But here is where it gets

23

a little strange.

The rock tribe decided to help the plant tribe in easing man's pain. Now the head of the rock tribe was Quartz. The myth tells us that there is an intimate relation between quartz and tobacco: " The Quartz crystal put his arm around *his brother tobacco* and said 'I will be the sacred mineral . . .'"

Now what relationship can a rock possibly have with a plant, especially in this case? Why does quartz (a rock) call tobacco (a plant) brother? It seems a little strange but here is where modern science helps us out.

It turns out that the Indian myths were precise in a very scientific way. Tobacco happens to be possibly the biggest silica accumulator on the earth. What is silica? Just another name for quartz. A silica accumulator is a plant that attracts silica from the soil more than your average plant. These plants love this mineral called silica and tobacco is a big silica accumulator, maybe the biggest.

It is so much a part of the plant that researchers have discovered that silica is even embedded into the very leaf structure in tiny granules called phytoliths. Here is what the researchers found regarding silica: "Examination of the tobacco leaves under a dissecting microscope (x32) revealed particles embedded in the surface, despite previous ultrasonic and mechanical removal of surface dust." The researchers went on to conclude that silica must be a "part of the leaf structure as the result of metabolic processes of the plant itself." (Journal of the American Dental Association March 1995)

OK. So what? The Indians were right about silica being in the tobacco plant. What does that matter?

It matters because silica is necessary for the body and the brain. Modern science has uncovered the role

25

of silica in structural formaton of bone, skin and hair .
. . but it doesn't stop there. It seems the Indian myth
has some more to say about silica as to its function.

The myth goes on with quartz saying some rather
interesting things about its abilities to help the human
race. "I will be the sacred mineral. I will heal the mind."

Silica has something to do with the mind according to Indian myth. Does science back this up?

It does. Doctor Allen Gaby reported on an interesting study in France that was published in the
American Journal of Clinical Nutrition (2005;81:897–902)
in which silica intake played a primary role in cognitive behavior. Close to 8,000 French women over the
age of 75 years old participated. At the beginning of
the study the women were assessed as to how much silica was being taken in their diet and then tests were
given. Gaby reports, "Women with lower intakes of

silica were found to perform worse on cognitive function tests, compared with women whose silica intake from drinking water was higher."

Follow ups were done on some of the women for up to seven years and Gaby concluded that, "During the follow-up period, women with lower intake of silica were at increased risk of developing Alzheimer's disease; those who developed Alzheimer's disease were nearly three times as likely to have a low silica intake from drinking water (4 mg per day or less)."

This should come as no surprise because about 30 years before this trial, another scientist, Edith Carlyle, noted that the brain was practically made of silica. In the text *Silicon Biochemistry* she noted that certain areas of the rat brain have a higher degree of silicon concentration than other areas from dietary uptake. She states, "regional concentrations of silicon varied. For instance, in the hippocampus,

27

caudate and lentiform nucleus, silicon concentrations were greater than in the other nine regions examined. It appeared as if silicon had some function in the brain."(pg.176)

According to scientists there is very little difference between a rat brain and a human brain. Rodents share more than just the reward pathway with humans. The entire set-up of the brain is nearly identical. Both use the same neurotransmitters and receptors, the same proteins for synaptic vesicle release and recycling, and similar signaling mechanisms.

But what is interesting about Carlyle's discovery was *where* the silicon was concentrated. The hippocampus for instance, is noted for being the primary area where memory is stored in the brain. And memory is exactly the problem in dementias of the brain such as Alzheimers disease.

Oh, and we must not forget the role that silicon

plays in our society— computer memory. Hmmm .
. . seems like the Indian myths were on to something when the Quartz crystal also says, "I will *record*
their spiritual history . . ." Record? Modern science
has shown us that this is silicons primary function.
Our whole society is based on this mineral record-
ing and storing knowledge. From computers to cell
phones and tons of other devices there is one mineral
responsible for holding data— silicon. Same goes in
the human brain.

Speaking of Alzheimers . . . researchers seem
to notice that there is a great disproportion between
aluminum and silicon in these patients. There is more
aluminum then silica. It turns out that aluminum as
a mineral has the ability to chemically push silica out
from regions that it is concentrated in.

It turns out that the Indian myth is kind of scary
now doesn't it? Though it is presented in non-scientific

language it seems that the things it touches on have support in modern science.

But there is another surprise that involves this mineral. Though our civilization is based on this mineral, it seems that it has been removed from our food supply. Silica is concentrated in certain foods and one of them happens to be cereal grains. The fibrous region of all grains is a veritable container of silica. But guess what was removed from grains beginning in the early 20th century? The fibrous region called the bran was removed in wide-scale industrial processing techniques. What is left is the endosperm which white bread is made from.

The 20th century could be called the white bread century because most of the populations of the earth ate this product. But now you must pay close attention.

Remember what Richter found out about an animal when it has a deficiency of a nutrient? It will seek this nutrient out and acquire it even if it is in a non-food. And that is precisely what cigarette smokers do. Since silica has been stripped from our food supply on a massive scale the body will try to acquire this nutrient in some form any form even if it is a non-food.

And if you've been paying attention in this chapter you know what non-food has high amounts of silica— TOBACCO.

It follows that if silica is replaced in the diet through certain foods and/or supplements one thing will happen. Like magic, the desire to smoke cigarettes will completely vanish! A good enough reason to call it the Magic Mineral.

4

Smoking Is History

If you are a smoker— picture this: Tomorrow you light up a cigarette and you take a puff. Then something happens that hasn't happened since the very first time you smoked a cigarette— you gag and cough, the taste is so bad.

Later that day, someone else lights up and a strange feeling of disgust comes over you because you can't stand the smell of the smoke. You think to yourself, 'What the heck is happening to me?'

But wait . . . this gets even better. That night you get a phone call from your friend and usually this is the time that you light up and smoke like a chimney. Half way through the conversation you look down at your hands and you think to yourself, 'Why aren't I holding a cigarette?'

The next day the strangest of all things happens to you and this one tops them all. Just thinking about a cigarette disgusts you. Two days ago you were smoking a pack a day and now you can't even bear to think about it— you even shudder.

How can this come about?

The answer is silica . . .

The above scenario is not fiction. This was exactly my experience and the experience of many others who quit smoking— without trying.

Of course the first time this happened to me I didn't know what was going on— I was mystified even more so than friends and co-workers who noticed. People around me thought I was *trying* to quit but I definitely was not— I thoroughly enjoyed smoking and had no intentions of quitting.

Still, everyone around me persisted in saying that I was *trying* to quit. I tried to explain that I didn't *feel* like smoking. There is a world of difference between the two. Eventually I started smoking again about a year later. The craving for cigarettes came back and so I smoked for about five more years— a pack a day.

And then *it* happenend again . . . I couldn't stand the sight or smell of cigarettes! What was going on here? Again the criticism came that I was trying to quit or that I was secretly taking a nicotine gum or some such thing. This time I resumed smoking a few months later. The craving came back and so I smoked.

But this phenomenon of quitting without trying occurred several times to me over the years. But what I didn't know then I fully realize now:

When I stopped smoking without trying I didn't know that I was consuming a particular silica rich food— regularly.

Everytime that I started eating this particular silica rich food— I would stop smoking. And I was a pack a day smoker. After realizing that it was due to silica consumption, I could turn the desire for cigarettes on and off like a switch.

Consume the silica rich food— desire for smoking gone.

Stop eating the silica rich food— desire for smoking comes back within days.

So what was that particular food that was responsible for this?

The humble cucumber.

The cucumber is a silica vegetable and considered a silica accumulator in the plant kingdom. Not only that but it contains other vitamins and minerals that we need. Whenever I quit smoking, it always corresponded to the intake of this vegetable. During these times I was eating anywhere from two to four cucumbers a day and almost overnight I could not stand the taste or the thought of cigarette smoking. But why does this occur?

When I fed my body silica from a whole food source in the right amounts, my body didn't

need or crave the silica from the tobacco. I fed the hunger of the cell, for silica, through a natural food rather than from a nonfood such as tobacco.

Well, eventually these 'cucumber kicks' would end and I eventually would find myself smoking again. I never put two and two together because I didn't realize the connection until years later.

When I finally found out that silica is the 'missing factor' in cigarette smoking I experimented with supplements and other foods and here is what I found.

Silica is hard to come by— at least in food.

Silica is in many foods but not in as great amounts or as concentrated as in the cucumber. Nothing rivals the cucumber because it is a silica accumulator.

Grains are a rich source of silica— but not in our civilization. Silica resides in the fibrous portion of the grain but our civilization has stripped fiber from the grain. Fiber is a carrier of silica (as is tobacco) and we are a fiberless civilization due to widespread refining processes. But this can explain how some people quit because they adopt a healthier lifestyle by eating fiber rich foods and eating better foods in general.

If the body does not have silica in a food source it will turn to a nonfood source such as tobacco. This is the story of the 20th century and even the early part of the 21st. Our cells are starving for this mineral and the industrial refining of grains is keeping it away from us. As I've said before, the 20th century should be known as the white bread century. And what did people do for their silica? Before the Surgeon Generals report came out in 1965 the smoking rate in America was estimated to be well over 50%. It's simple . . . the body needs a source of silica and it doesn't matter where it comes from. Silica was taken out of a staple food source (grains) in the 20th century, so people turned to another source in the 20th century . . . tobacco.

In other words, what I am saying is that if we had real grains and real grain products, such as whole grain sprouted bread, in the 20th century, there would not have been a smoking problem to speak of.

There are three ways to incorporate silica into the diet in order to quit smoking . . .

1) Food

2) Supplements

3) Food and supplements combined

FOOD ONLY

An example of the food only method comes from an individual who bought my first book to help her husband to quit smoking.

Vera D. had a bad experience when her husband tried to quit smoking 10 years previously. Because, as explained in detail in my first book, you CAN

NOT quit silica. Your body is like a machine that demands this mineral. If you 'quit' one source it WILL CHOOSE another source. And the choice that people make when they quit, unfortunately, is a very bad one— sugar. This is also explained in my book, how sugar contains a residue, a minute amount of silica. What does this mean for the person choosing this source that has very little silica? Much more of this source must be consumed.

And this is exactly what happens. In the case of Vera D.'s husband, he consumed more sugar and refined grains throughout the day then he ever had before. By the next year he developed a complication from consuming this silica source— diabetes. This and many other complications such as weight gain and heart disease are associated with this silica source called sugar.

Needless to say her husband resumed smoking and

never looked back on trying to quit smoking until Vera D. bought the book. She read about the silica sources and decided to try the cucumber diet. But there was one catch— her husband didn't realize that it was for the purpose of quitting smoking. So it was sort of like a single-blind study. She just proposed the cucumber diet as a healthy alternative to help his diabetes. The issue of cucumbers to quit smoking was never brought up to her husband who, by the way, was a smoker for over 40 years.

You must keep in mind that her husband ate his normal diet except for the addition of cucumbers as a snack and side-dish, rather than his sugary snacks or refined grains like white bread.

This was her plan of attack . . .

Four cucumbers spread out throughout the day in various ways and forms. I have personally quit on less per day but for some reason she chose four.

Perhaps it was because she thought that he was a long time smoker and he really needed some serious silica saturation in order to quit. For whatever reason, in her case, she judged correctly . . . because it worked.

In the morning she put one cucumber and various other greens into a blender. This was her husbands first cucumber of the day. By the way, the best approach is to have some form of silica rich product in the morning as soon as you wake up.

The second cucumber was a side dish to his lunch which was usually a sandwich.

The third cucumber was a part of the dinner salad which was had every night.

The fourth cucumber was his late night snack between ten and twelve o'clock.

All of these cucumbers had the skin still on them. This is important because the silica resides in the skin so DO NOT PEEL the skin. In fact this goes for all

41

fruits and vegetables— think skin.

That first week his cigarette smoking began to wane. A pack a day smoker went to half a pack in two days and for the few days after that, barely five a day. By the end of the week he was not smoking.

And now for the hilarious part. At the beginning of the second week he proudly announced that he had quit smoking. Now, keep in mind that this had not entered his head for at least ten years but now he believed that he could 'do it' on his own. And he had no idea that the cucumbers served a different purpose than he thought— and he still doesn't have any idea about the cucumbers being the cause of his quitting.

For whatever reason or motive that she chose the stealth method, it was still clearly a success because 8 months later, at the time of this book being published, her husband is still smoke free.

But the fascinating part of all this is that her husband doesn't have the urges and he doesn't have the nervousness and mood swings that he had the first time he tried to quit.

As a side note Vera D., after seeing the success her husband was having, decided to use the same stealth technique with her son who was somewhat of a casual smoker— about a pack of cigarettes every few days to a week. She managed to 'sneak' in two cucumbers a day into his diet and he soon 'decided to quit smoking.' Unbeknownst to him, it was the silica in the cucumber that brought him to this 'decision.'

I have tried many different foods that have high silica content but the two with the biggest punch are:

1) Cucumbers

2) Whole Grain Sprouted bread

Since we have talked about cucumbers I would like to talk about what happened when I tried sliced bread which was sprouted.

The whole issue of bread is talked about in the other book so I won't get into it here except to say one thing: Sprouted whole grain bread will yield more of a particular nutrient for absorption in the body than regular whole grain bread.

The reason sprouted bread works to stop cravings for tobacco is because it has two special nutrients which tobacco also has— nicotinic acid and silica.

Five pieces of toasted sprouted bread with butter throughout the day made all cigarette cravings go away. Please keep in mind that I did this just to prove a point to myself that just one silica rich food could do the trick— I wanted to isolate each silica rich food and see what its abilities were. The key was starting out with two toasted pieces of sprouted bread right away in the morning. Then, several hours later another snack of two toasted pieces with butter. Late at night I would have another piece the same way. After a week, three or four slices toasted with butter did the trick. But why did I make sure they were toasted with butter?

Saturated fats, such as real butter and animal fat, are necessary for mineral absorption. Dr. Weston Price theorized about this almost a century ago and modern science has borne out his theory. In the International Journal of Sport Nutrition and Exercise Nutrition, a study was published in June 2001 issue which proved saturated fats, in distinction to unsaturated fats, have an important role in mineral absorption and retention in the human body. The study was conducted amongst athletes and what the researchers found was that the higher the poly-unsaturated fat consumption, the higher the loss of minerals which resulted in reduced endurance performance. The athletes that were on saturated fats were far more able to utilize and retain minerals. In other words, no saturated fat— no mineral absorption.

This applies to silica as well. For instance when I would have toast with no butter it was not as effective as toast with butter. Or if I had sandwiches with the sprouted bread— this also was not as effective as toast with butter.

SUPPLEMENTS ONLY

Mike L. did not like cucumbers and did not really want to change his dietary habits to incorporate silica into his diet. So he went the supplements route. As explained in my first book he chose silica supplements that were from a vegetal source— ultimately derived from a plant. The silica supplement was an extraction of silica from the horsetail herb— it was not strictly a horsetail herb extract. The horsetail herb is a plant that is possibly the richest in silica but in my first book I did not recommend this herb because of the side effects associated with it; so he took the supplement that extracts the silica from this herb. There are other forms such as ortho-silicic acid which claims to be the most bio-available but I do not have any experience with this form up to this pont in time. The other source is silica obtained from marine-derived Red Algae Powder (Lithothamnium coralloides). It is marketed by a company which calls it 'oceanic silica.' In my experience this form is also very effective.

So what we have is three forms

1) Silica derived from the horsetail herb

2) Silica derived from marine algae

3) Ortho-silicic acid

Anyway, Mike L. decided to take eight capsules a day (silica derived from horsetail herb) spread out throughout the day starting out with two in the morning. Mike L. was a pack of day smoker for over twenty years and by the second day of supplementation he was smoking four cigarettes but as he said they were 'half smoked'— he couldn't finish them. By the third day he had no cravings except for maybe one or two cigarettes at stressful times and these were 'always at work.' But keep in mind, Mike L., for some reason, was not following the advice of the book completely as we shall see.

By the second week he lowered the amounts to four capsules a day because, to him, 'it was a hassle taking those capsules.' He wanted as little intrusion as possible, from his non-smoking regimen, into his daily life. It still worked because he had developed a saturation of the silica.

At the end of the first month he was relatively smoke free and craving free except for an occassional cigarette or two. These one or two cigarettes were always during the work week but other than that he had no desire or cravings like he had for the last twenty years.

An interesting thing happened with Mike L.— according to him 'this was just too easy.' He began to think that the silica was just a placebo, that it was all just a psychological effect. So he stopped the silica and decided he was just going to use 'will-power' since he thought the silica was just a placebo.

But you can't quit silica, as Mike L. soon found out. Within days the 'will-power' method failed and he was back to smoking a pack a day.

A few months went by and all the while he wondered about the silica and read my first book again. After reading it and understanding the science behind it, he became convinced that cigarette smoking was due to a deficiency of the Magic Mineral— silica.

So he began the silica supplementation (this second time happened to be with the oceanic silica, as none other was available) but he decided he wanted to do away with those occassional one or two cigarettes

49

that he would smoke when he quit the last time with silica. Reading my book more carefully the second time, he understood that silica works in conjunction with nicotinic acid or vitamin B-3— this is what he ignored the first time. As my book explains, this vitamin is related to nicotine. For example, it is well known among chemists and biochemists that when nicotine is oxidized it becomes nicotinic acid which is another name for B-3. Whether this occurs in the body or not is taken up in my first book, so we will just leave it at that for now.

But Mike L. found that when he consistently supplemented with both silica and vitamin B-3 the problem of those 'occassional one or two cigarettes' was gone. He got to the point where even thinking about a cigarette made him cringe. With regular silica and B-3 supplementation he has not looked back and has not felt the slightest cravings. After the initial saturation stage, in which he took eight capsules a day along with four B-Complex for about a week, he weened down to four silica capsules a day and two to three B-Complex which is his regular regimen until this day.

A word must be said about the type of B vitamin that Mike L. used. It was a B Complex whole food derived capsule. This is the best form of vitamin to take because it will be absorbed by the body far better than any chemicalized vitamin. It was recommended to him to take a B-Complex rather than just B-3. The B-Complex contains all of the B vitamins, including B-3, which act synergistically with one another for a more powerful effect. It is up to you. Read the first book for more information.

FOOD AND SUPPLEMENTS COMBINED

Food alone is extremely effective but food plus supplements really puts it over the top!

One time I decided to add the supplements to the

51

sprouted bread method.

Each time I had sprouted bread (toasted with butter!) I would supplement with two capsules of silica (oceanic silica) and one B Complex. The first day by the end of the day ALL DESIRE FOR SMOKING WAS GONE. I kept this pace for a week and then was able to pick and choose what I wanted to with silica supplements and/or foods.

Let your creativity come in here and come up with ways to incorporate both cucumbers and sprouted bread and supplements and even other silica rich foods.

You can even put herbal supplements into the mix if you want. So many herbal concoctions are offered on the market for smoking cessation and it is really all ridiculous. Why? Because most of the herbs serve absolutely NO PURPOSE in smoking cessation!

How can I be sure of this? Because they are not silica rich herbs. Sometimes the herbal smoking concoctions do carry a silica rich herb and this is why they may 'work.' But they would be way more effective if they emphasized the silica rich herbs. You don't need to spend unnecessary money for unnecessary herbs. The silica rich herbs to incorporate would be:

1) Horsetail

2) Oat straw

3) Sarsaparilla root

4) Licorice root

5) Echinacinae

You could eat a silica food with a silica supplement and then a couple hours later, a silica herb. Then a different silica food followed a couple hours later with a supplement and so and so on . . .

Also there is a homeopathic remedy that could be incorporated into the mix which is known as *lobelia*. This is also known as Indian tobacco. I wonder what mineral this plant has traces of ?

The TWO most important things to remember on a silica rich diet?

1) REGULARITY— just like you regularly smoked, for the first week you must conscientiously supply silica and B-3 to your cells at regular intervals

2) DO NOT TRY TO STOP SMOKING— In fact I smoked whenever I felt it but what I found was that the more I saturated my body with these two nutrients the feeling for smoking just simply was not there. There is absolutely no desire to smoke because you are feeding yourself the two things that the cigarette was giving you without all those other dangerous chemicals the cigarette has.

And believe me this happens FAST. We are talking about hours not days. But it depended on the zeal with which I fed these two nutrients to my body. When I thought about it, I regularly smoked throughout the day. This meant that I had to regularly feed my body these two nutrients throughout the day.

In all three methods, the results were immediate—hours not days. But I concentrated on feeding myself those two nutrients through food and/or supplement. With the combination method I stopped taking the supplements within about a week. I didn't need them. I saturated my body with silica through food and supplements that I developed a saturation point— so after about a week I just ate silica rich foods. No need for the supplements. It truly is amazing how I went from one extreme to the other. From craving cigarettes to becoming a non-smoking advocate berating everyone who smoked and complaining about how aweful the smell was to others that were smoking. A week before this I was puffing away to my hearts content.

But again, whenever I tried one of these three

methods I DID NOT TRY TO STOP SMOKING. By focusing on silica foods and supplements it came naturally and it came fast.

And there's NO SUCH THING as FALLING OFF THE WAGON if you start smoking again. You are just trading your source of silica from a healthy one (silica foods and supplements) to one that has bad side effects (tobacco with all the bad chemicals in it). Now that you have the knowledge, you understand that there is no such thing as addiction to cigarettes because it is all about the Magic Mineral, silica.

SMOKING IS HISTORY